"Juicing for Fatty Liver"

Revitalize your Liver with Nourishing Fruit Extracts for Enhanced Wellness

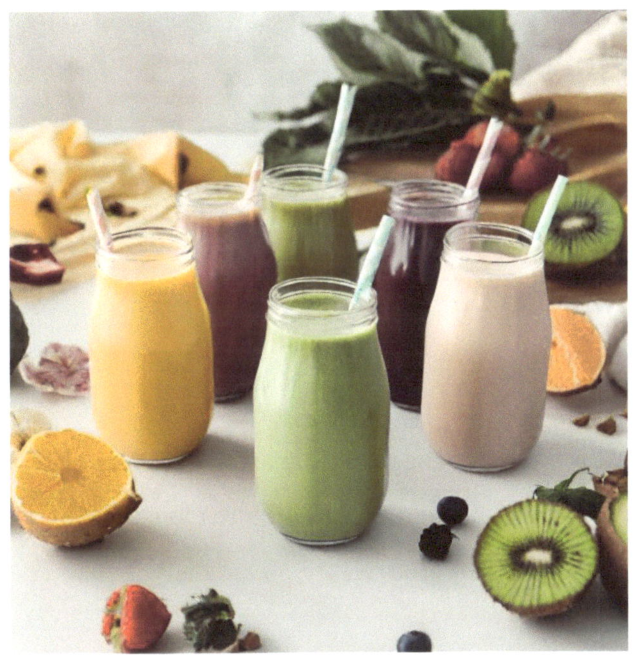

Catherine D Crisp

Disclaimer

The information in the book is based on personal research and experience. The author advises readers to consult with their healthcare provider before making any dietary changes

For more information or to contact the author, please email: catherinecrispnutrition@gmail.com

TABLE OF CONTENTS

CONCLUSION: JUICING FOR FATTY LIVER – A PATH TOWARDS HEALTH

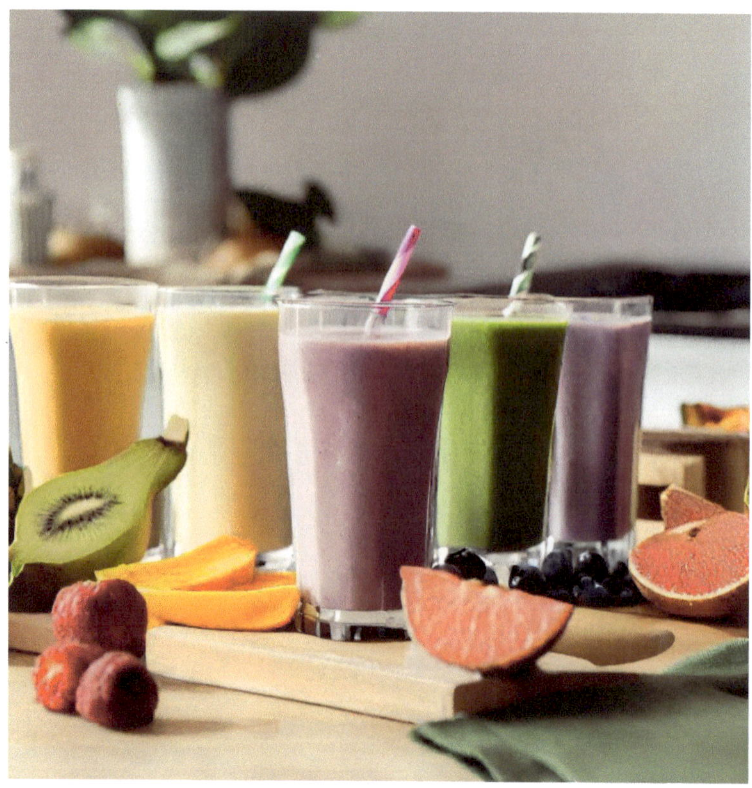

Why I'm Writing This Book

Dear friend. I am writing this book with a profound sense of purpose, driven by a deeply emotional connection to a cause that has touched my heart and soul. Fatty liver disease, a silent yet insidious condition, has affected countless lives, including that of my dear friend Alex. Witnessing her struggle and the shock of her diagnosis ignited a fire within me, compelling me to take action and make a difference.

Alex's life took an unexpected turn in her early thirties when she received a diagnosis that sent shockwaves through her world: **fatty liver disease.** It was a diagnosis she never saw coming, a disease she associated with older individuals or those who had indulged in unhealthy habits for years. Yet, there she was, sitting in the doctor's office, grappling with a reality she couldn't ignore.

The news hit her like a ton of bricks. The thought of her liver, one of the most vital organs in her body, slowly succumbing to fat infiltration was terrifying. She knew she had to take action, and fast.

Almost losing my uncle to heart problems nearly a decade ago, turned me into a health enthusiast, as I searched for alternative treatments for his condition. I detail that experience in my book: **Heart Healthy Cooking with DASH: 215 Delicious Recipes for Managing High Blood Pressure Naturally.**

I recently delved into the world of juicing, believing in its power to heal the body from the inside out. When I learned about Alex's diagnosis, I knew I had to share what I had discovered.

The very next day, I invited Alex over and laid out my plan. I explained how specific fruits and vegetables, when juiced together, could work wonders for the liver.

Alex, though initially skeptical, saw the hope in my eyes and decided to give it a shot. She had nothing to lose and everything to gain. We started small, crafting basic liver-friendly juices that were not only nutritious but surprisingly delicious. We mixed kale, spinach, apples, and a dash of lemon juice, creating a vibrant green elixir that became a daily ritual.

In 14 short days, Alex began to notice changes in her health. The fatigue that had once gripped her began to loosen its hold. Her energy levels soared, and the constant discomfort in her abdomen began to subside. She could feel her body healing from the inside out, one sip at a time.

As our journey continued, Alex became more adventurous with her juices. She experimented with different combinations, incorporating ingredients like beets, ginger, and turmeric to enhance liver detoxification. Her kitchen turned into a laboratory of health, a place where she mixed and matched vibrant colors and flavors to create concoctions that nourished her ailing liver.

The next month, Alex returned to her doctor for a check-up, her heart pounding with anticipation. The results were nothing short of astonishing. Her liver enzymes had improved significantly, and her doctor couldn't believe the transformation. Alex's liver was on its way to recovery. Tears welled up in my friend's eyes as she hugged me tightly. She had found a path to healing, a path she hadn't known existed, and it was all thanks to our belief in the power of juicing for liver health.

The emotional turmoil that Alex and her loved ones endured left an indelible mark on my conscience. It was a wake-up call, a stark reminder of how fragile our health can be and how imperative it is to prioritize our well-being. It is for this reason I wrote this guide; to empower you, dear friend, with the tools and understanding needed to combat fatty liver disease. In this guide, I share the transformative potential of juicing, a healing method that can rejuvenate your liver and entire being. I hope that through these pages, you will find inspiration, support, and the knowledge required to take control of your health.

Introduction

Welcome to "Juicing for Fatty Liver: Revitalize your Liver with Nourishing Fruit Extracts for Enhanced Wellness." This book's goal is to give a complete guide for beginners on how juicing may help with liver health and overall well-being.

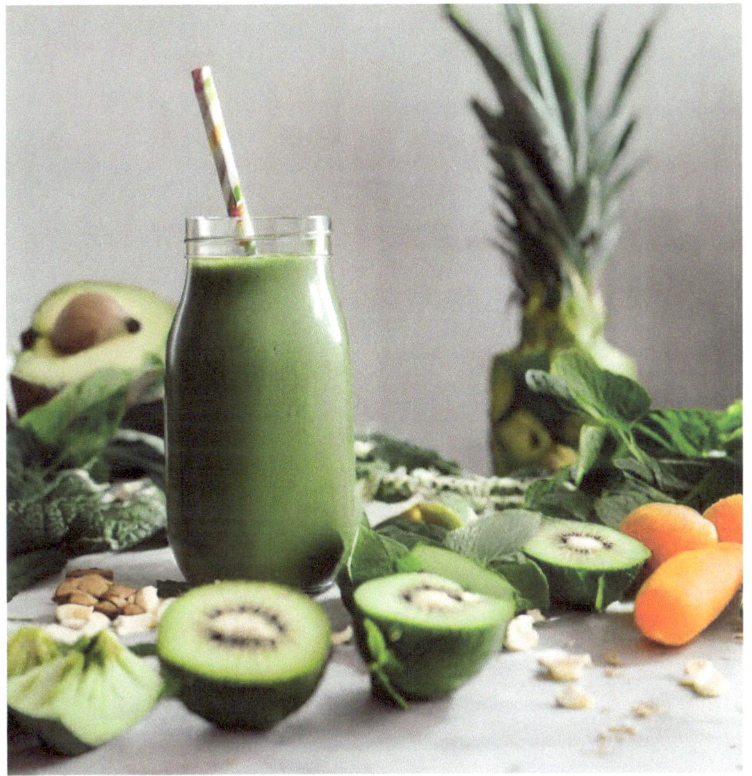

Your liver is essential to your general health since it aids in digestion, cleansing, and metabolism. The liver's capacity to operate properly may be affected when it is burdened by factors such as poor dietary choices, excessive alcohol intake, or certain medical diseases such as fatty liver disease.

Juicing, or extracting the juice from fruits and vegetables, can be a valuable tool for supporting and improving liver function. We can supply critical nutrients, antioxidants, and enzymes to our liver in a handy and readily digested manner by ingesting freshly extracted juices.

This book will teach you about the various advantages of juicing for fatty liver. We'll look at how juices can provide powerful antioxidants that protect the liver from free radicals and promote recovery. Juicing can also help reduce inflammation, aid in weight reduction, improve digestion, and increase energy levels. You will also learn practical recommendations on picking the ideal fruits and vegetables for liver health, as well as information on how to properly prepare and store your juices, to make juicing simple and successful for you.

You'll find a range of tasty juice recipes throughout the chapters that are particularly designed to nourish and improve your liver. These drinks will incorporate a variety of fruits, vegetables, and herbs that are beneficial to the liver. They are easy to create and require only a few ingredients, making them ideal for even complete beginners.

It is crucial to highlight that this book is for educational purposes and should not be used as a substitute for medical advice. Please speak with a healthcare practitioner before making any substantial changes to your diet or lifestyle if you have particular liver-related concerns or medical issues.

So, let's start juicing and unlock the potential for a healthy liver and a happier, more vibrant you!

What exactly is Fatty Liver Disease?

Our liver is a vital organ that processes nutrition, removes toxins from our bodies, and produces bile to facilitate digestion. Fatty liver disease is characterized by an abnormal accumulation of fat in the liver.

A poor diet heavy in sugar and saturated fats, excessive alcohol use, obesity, certain medicines, or even genetic susceptibility can all contribute to excess fat. When fat accumulates in the liver cells, it can cause inflammation and damage, impairing the liver's capacity to function normally.

Fatty liver disease is classified into two types: alcoholic fatty liver disease and non-alcoholic fatty liver disease (NAFLD). Excessive alcohol intake causes alcoholic fatty liver disease, whereas NAFLD is connected with variables such as obesity, insulin resistance, elevated blood sugar levels, and other metabolic diseases.

Fatty liver disease is sometimes referred to be a silent illness since it may not manifest any symptoms in the early stages. However, if the condition advances, weariness, stomach pain, jaundice (yellowing of the skin and eyes), and abdominal swelling may ensue. As a result, addressing fatty liver disease early on is critical to preventing additional liver damage.

The good news is that fatty liver disease can typically be controlled, if not reversed, with lifestyle adjustments such as dietary alterations. This is where juicing may help significantly improve and maintain liver health.

We can improve liver function and prevent fat formation by introducing fresh, nutrient-rich fruit extracts into our diet. Fruit juices nourish our liver with vital vitamins, minerals, antioxidants, and enzymes that promote healing, reduce inflammation, and maintain its general health.

It is important to note, however, that while juicing can be a fantastic tool for liver health, it is not a replacement for medical counsel. If you feel you have fatty liver disease or any other liver-related issues, you should see a doctor for a correct diagnosis and treatment.

The Importance of Nutrition in the Management of Fatty Liver Disease

When it comes to fatty liver disease, the food we consume has a huge impact on whether or not our liver heals. Nutritional support is critical for controlling this illness and increasing liver function.

A nutritious diet can aid in the reduction of fat buildup in the liver, the reduction of inflammation, and the support of the liver's capacity to function effectively. It can also aid in the management of underlying diseases such as obesity and insulin resistance, which are frequently associated with fatty liver disease.

So, what foods should we eat to assist our liver? For starters, nutritious fruits! Fruits are high in vitamins, minerals, antioxidants, and fiber, all of which are good for our liver health. They can help minimize oxidative stress, inflammation, and enhance liver cell regeneration.

Natural fruit juice may be a quick and tasty method to get these essential nutrients into our diet. We may access the concentrated benefits of a variety of fruits in an easily edible form by extracting the juices from them. Apples, berries, citrus fruits, pineapples, and grapes are very good for your liver. These fruits are high in antioxidants, which help protect the liver from free radical damage.

In this book, you will learn important information, practical ideas, and tasty juicing recipes that are particularly meant to nourish and enhance the health of your liver

The Advantages of Juicing for Liver Health

Juicing is the process of extracting the juice from fresh fruits and vegetables in order to provide you with a concentrated dose of their nutrients. Juicing has been shown to be quite good to our liver!

For starters, juicing can help you to consume more fruits and vegetables in a handy and readily digested manner. This means you can acquire a range of vitamins, minerals, and antioxidants that are needed for liver function in one dose. Juicing can also assist enhance hydration, which is crucial for liver function. A well-hydrated liver can effectively remove poisons and waste from our bodies.

Juicing is also an excellent method to include more veggies into our diet, such as carrots, beets, and leafy greens. These vegetables are high in vital nutrients like vitamin C, beta-carotene, and folate, which help improve the general health of our liver.

Another advantage of juicing is that it helps us consume more fiber. Although the juicing process eliminates some fiber, we may acquire a sufficient quantity by including pulp or adding fiber-rich products such as chia seeds to our juice. Fiber aids in the promotion of good digestion, the regulation of blood sugar levels, and the general functioning of our liver.

Juicing is also a delightful and refreshing method to consume fruits and vegetables, making it simpler to keep to a balanced eating plan. It allows us to experiment with diverse flavors and combinations, guaranteeing that our juices never get boring.

However, understand that juicing should not be used in place of complete fruits and vegetables. Whole meals give additional critical minerals and fiber that juicing may not. Juicing should be viewed as a supplement to a healthy diet.

In this guide, you will discover a variety of healthy and simple juice recipes that are particularly tailored to assist your liver health.

Kindly speak with your doctor or healthcare professional to get specific counsel, especially if you have any underlying health concerns.

Juicing Recipes for Your Liver Health

In this chapter, we'll dive right into the main course of our journey: making your liver-boosting juices.

Here, we'll look at the art and science of creating juices that are particularly designed to help your liver heal. Each recipe is a carefully selected combination of nature's best ingredients, designed to provide your body with the nutrition it requires. You'll be feeding your liver one glass at a time from the minute you take your first drink.

So be ready for a fascinating adventure through a world of flavors and colors.

1. Beet and Berry Blast Smoothie

This delectable smoothie is high in antioxidants and anti-inflammatory ingredients, which can benefit liver function. Betains, which are abundant in beets, have been found to benefit liver function.

Ingredients:

- 1 small beet, peeled and sliced

- 1 cup mixed berries (blueberries, raspberries, strawberries)

- ½ banana

- 1 cup unsweetened almond milk

- 1 tbsp honey

Instructions:

1. Blend the beet and berries in a blender until finely chopped.

2. Add the remaining ingredients and blend until smooth.

3. Serve immediately.

2. Green Detox Smoothie

This pleasant and colorful green smoothie will detoxify your liver. This smoothie is high in fiber, vitamins, and minerals since it contains leafy greens and citrus fruits.

Ingredients:

- 2 cups spinach

- 1 small cucumber, chopped

- 1 apple, chopped

- ½ avocado

- 1 cup orange juice

- 1 tsp grated ginger

Instructions:

1. Blend all the ingredients together until smooth.

2. Pour into a glass and enjoy!

3. Pineapple and Turmeric Smoothie

Pineapple contains bromelain, an enzyme with anti-inflammatory effects and the ability to ease digestion. Turmeric has anti-inflammatory properties and can help with liver health.

Ingredients:

- 1 cup pineapple chunks

- ½ banana

- 1 cup unsweetened coconut milk

- 1 tbsp honey

- ½ tsp turmeric powder

Instructions:

1. Place all ingredients in a blender and blend until smooth.

2. Pour into a glass and enjoy!

4. Carrot and Ginger Smoothie

Carrots are high in beta-carotene, a potent antioxidant that can help protect the liver. Ginger has anti-inflammatory properties and can aid digestion.

Ingredients:

- 2 carrots, chopped

- ½ banana

- ½ inch fresh ginger, grated

- 1 cup unsweetened almond milk

- 1 tbsp honey

Instructions:

1. Blend all the ingredients together until smooth.

2. Pour into a glass and enjoy!

<u>**5. Berry and Coconut Smoothie**</u>

This smoothie is high in antioxidants and good fats, which can aid in inflammation reduction and liver health.

Ingredients:

- 1 cup mixed berries (strawberries, raspberries, blueberries)

- 1 small banana

- 1 cup unsweetened coconut milk

- 1 tbsp chia seeds

Instructions:

1. Blend the berries, banana, and coconut milk in a blender until smooth.

2. Stir in the chia seeds and let the smoothie sit for 5-10 minutes to thicken.

3. Pour into a glass and enjoy!

6. Mango and Lime Smoothie

Mangoes are high in vitamin C, which can help protect the liver from oxidative stress damage. Lime is high in vitamin C and might help with digestion.

Ingredients:

- 1 mango, peeled and chopped

- 1 small banana

- 1 cup unsweetened almond milk

- Juice of 1 lime

Instructions:

1. Blend all the ingredients together until smooth.

2. Pour into a glass and enjoy!

7. Blueberry and Almond Smoothie

Blueberries are high in flavonoids, which have antioxidant and anti-inflammatory properties that can help preserve the liver. Almonds are high in healthy fats and can aid to prevent inflammation.

Ingredients:

- 1 cup blueberries

- 1 small banana

- 1 cup unsweetened almond milk

- ¼ cup almonds

- 1 tsp honey

Instructions:

1. Blend all the ingredients together until smooth.

2. Pour into a glass and enjoy!

8. Apple and Cinnamon Smoothie

Apples are high in antioxidants and can aid in the reduction of inflammation. Cinnamon contains anti-inflammatory and antioxidant qualities that can benefit liver function.

Ingredients:

- 1 apple, chopped

- 1 small banana

- 1 cup unsweetened almond milk

- 1 tsp cinnamon powder

- 1 tsp honey

Instructions:

1. Blend all the ingredients together until smooth.

2. Pour into a glass and enjoy!

9. Kale and Pineapple Smoothie

Kale contains vitamins and minerals that can help the liver operate. Bromelain, an enzyme found in pineapple, helps aid digestion and decrease inflammation.

Ingredients:

- 2 cups kale

- 1 cup pineapple chunks

- 1 small banana

- 1 cup unsweetened coconut milk

- 1 tsp honey

Instructions:

1. Blend all the ingredients together until smooth.

2. Pour into a glass and enjoy!

<u>**10. Chocolate Avocado Smoothie**</u>

This smoothie is high in antioxidants, fiber, and healthy fats. Avocados and dark chocolate both contain antioxidants that can help protect the liver from harm.

Ingredients:

- ½ avocado

- 1 small banana

- 1 cup unsweetened almond milk

- 1 tbsp unsweetened cocoa powder

- 1 tsp honey

Instructions:

1. Blend all the ingredients together until smooth.

2. Pour into a glass and enjoy!

11. Pomegranate and Pear Smoothie

Pomegranate contains antioxidants and anti-inflammatory chemicals that can help preserve the liver. Pears are high in fiber and can help with digestion.

Ingredients:

- ½ cup pomegranate seeds

- 1 pear, chopped

- 1 small banana

- 1 cup unsweetened almond milk

Instructions:

1. Blend all the ingredients together until smooth.

2. Pour into a glass and enjoy!

12. Turmeric and Ginger Smoothie

Both turmeric and ginger contain anti-inflammatory and antioxidant qualities that can benefit liver function. This smoothie is ideal for decreasing inflammation and aiding digestion.

Ingredients:

- ½ inch fresh turmeric, grated

- ½ inch fresh ginger, grated

- 1 small banana

- 1 cup unsweetened almond milk

- 1 tsp honey

Instructions:

1. Blend all the ingredients together until smooth.

2. Pour into a glass and enjoy!

13. Spinach and Pineapple Smoothie

Spinach is high in elements that help the liver function, such as iron and folate. Bromelain, an enzyme found in pineapple, can help with digestion and inflammation.

Ingredients:

- 2 cups spinach

- 1 cup pineapple chunks

- 1 small banana

- 1 cup unsweetened coconut milk

- 1 tsp honey

Instructions:

1. Blend all the ingredients together until smooth.

2. Pour into a glass and enjoy!

14. Berry and Chia Smoothie

This smoothie is high in antioxidants, fiber, and omega-3 fatty acids. Chia seeds are high in fiber and can aid to relieve inflammation.

Ingredients:

- 1 cup mixed berries (strawberries, raspberries, blueberries)

- 1 small banana

- 1 cup unsweetened almond milk

- 2 tbsp chia seeds

- 1 tsp honey

Instructions:

1. Blend all the ingredients together until smooth.

2. Pour into a glass and enjoy!

15. Mango and Coconut Smoothie

Mangoes include elements that assist liver function, such as vitamin C and beta-carotene. Coconut contains medium-chain triglycerides, which can aid in inflammation reduction.

Ingredients:

- 1 mango, peeled and chopped

- 1 small banana

- 1 cup unsweetened coconut milk

- 1 tsp honey

Instructions:

1. Blend all the ingredients together until smooth.

2. Pour into a glass and enjoy!

16. Orange and Carrot Smoothie

Oranges are high in vitamin C, which can help protect the liver. Carrots are also high in elements that promote liver health, such as beta-carotene.

Ingredients:

- 2 oranges, peeled and segmented

- 2 carrots, chopped

- 1 small banana

- 1 cup unsweetened almond milk

Instructions:

1. Blend all the ingredients together until smooth.

2. Pour into a glass and enjoy!

<u>**17. Blueberry and Spinach Smoothie**</u>

Blueberries are high in antioxidants, which can help protect the liver. Iron and folate are two elements found in spinach that can help with liver function.

Ingredients:

- 1 cup blueberries

- 2 cups spinach

- 1 small banana

- 1 cup unsweetened almond milk

- 1 tsp honey

Instructions:

1. Blend all the ingredients together until smooth.

2. Pour into a glass and enjoy!

18. Green Apple and Kale Smoothie

Green apples are high in antioxidants, which can help protect the liver. Kale includes elements that help the liver function, such as folate and vitamin C.

Ingredients:

- 1 green apple, chopped

- 2 cups kale

- 1 small banana

- 1 cup unsweetened almond milk

- 1 tsp honey

Instructions:

1. Blend all the ingredients together until smooth.

2. Pour into a glass and enjoy!

19. Raspberry and Mango Smoothie

Raspberries are rich in antioxidants, which can protect the liver from damage. Mangoes contain nutrients that can support liver health, including vitamin C and beta-carotene.

Ingredients:

- 1 cup raspberries

- 1 mango, peeled and chopped

- 1 small banana

- 1 cup unsweetened almond milk

Instructions:

1. Blend all the ingredients together until smooth.

2. Pour into a glass and enjoy!

<u>**20. Vanilla and Almond Smoothie**</u>

This smoothie is a good source of fiber, antioxidants, and good fats. Almonds and vanilla are foods that reduce liver inflammation.

Ingredients:

- 1 cup frozen blueberries

- 1 peeled banana

- 1 cup unsweetened almond milk

- 1 tablespoon chia seeds

- 1 teaspoon honey (optional)

Instructions:

1. Blend all ingredients in a blender until smooth.

2. Serve and enjoy!

21. Turmeric Mango Smoothie

The anti-inflammatory turmeric is added to this fruity smoothie, which also contains frozen mango, unsweetened coconut milk, and a little honey for flavor.

Ingredients:

- 1 cup frozen mango chunks

- 1 teaspoon turmeric powder

- 1 tablespoon honey

- 1 cup unsweetened coconut milk

Instructions:

1. Add all ingredients to a blender and blend until smooth.

2. Add more coconut milk if necessary to achieve a desired consistency

3. Blend all ingredients in a blender until smooth.

22. Green Goddess Smoothie:

The nutrients that support the health of the liver are abundant in this smoothie.

Ingredients:

- 1 cup baby spinach

- 1 peeled banana

- 1/2 cucumber, peeled and diced

- 1 tablespoon grated ginger

- 1 cup coconut water

Instructions:

1. Combine all ingredients in a blender and blend until smooth.

2. Pour into a glass and enjoy!

23. Papaya and Pineapple Smoothie:

The enzymes in this smoothie aid to enhance liver function.

Ingredients:

- 1 cup diced papaya

- 1 cup diced pineapple

- 1 peeled banana

- 1 cup unsweetened almond milk

Instructions:

1. Blend all ingredients in a blender until smooth.

2. Pour into a glass and enjoy!

<u>**24. Avocado Lime Smoothie**</u>

Made with avocado, ice, fresh lime juice, unsweetened almond milk, and a dash of honey, this creamy smoothie is delicious. It's a revitalizing for the liver and a fulfilling way to begin the day!

Ingredients:

- 1 small avocado, pitted and peeled

- Juice of 1 lime

- 1 tablespoon honey

- 1 cup unsweetened almond milk

- Ice

Instructions:

1. Add all ingredients to a blender and blend until smooth.
2. Add more almond milk if necessary to achieve the desired consistency.

25. Berry-Licious Smoothie:

Antioxidants found in this smoothie are great for defending the liver.

Ingredients:

- 1 cup mixed berries (strawberries, raspberries, blueberries)

- 1 peeled banana

- 1 cup unsweetened almond milk

- 1 tablespoon chia seeds

Instructions:

1. Combine all ingredients in a blender and blend until smooth.

2. Pour into a glass and enjoy!

Bonus Chapter: Unlocking the Healing Power of Smoothies for Cancer Management

Just as juicing has been shown to be a powerful aid for healing, the appropriate smoothie recipes can help individuals dealing with cancer. While we do not claim to have a miraculous cure for cancer, we think that nature's bounty, in the form of thoughtfully produced smoothies, may bring much-needed sustenance and solace throughout this difficult journey.

On the following pages, you'll find ten unique and meticulously prepared smoothie recipes, all of which are packed with cancer-fighting nutrients. These meals are about more than simply flavor; they are about empowerment and perseverance. We'll look at how various fruits, veggies, and superfoods might improve your general health and compliment your cancer treatment strategy.

1. Green Tea Berry Smoothie:

Green tea is high in antioxidants and may help prevent cancer, whereas berries are high in vitamins and antioxidants that fight cancer.

Ingredients:

- 1 cup frozen mixed berries

- 1/2 banana

- 1/2 cup brewed green tea, cooled

- 1/2 cup unsweetened almond milk

Instructions:

Add all ingredients to a blender and blend until smooth.

2. Mango Turmeric Smoothie:

This smoothie contains anti-inflammatory components that may aid in the reduction of inflammation in the body, which is frequently linked to cancer.

Ingredients:

- 1 cup frozen mango chunks

- 1 teaspoon turmeric powder

- 1/2 teaspoon ground ginger

- 1/2 cup unsweetened almond milk

- 1/2 cup water

Instructions:

Add all ingredients to a blender and blend until smooth.

3. Strawberry Basil Smoothie:

Strawberries are high in vitamin C and antioxidants, which may help prevent cancer, while basil has anti-inflammatory and cancer-fighting effects.

Ingredients:

- 1 cup frozen strawberries

- 1/4 cup fresh basil leaves

- 1/2 banana

- 1/2 cup unsweetened almond milk

Instructions:

Add all ingredients to a blender and blend until smooth.

<u>**4. Pineapple Ginger Smoothie:**</u>

Pineapple contains bromelain, an enzyme with anti-inflammatory qualities that may help lower the incidence of cancer, while ginger has been demonstrated to have anti-cancer effects.

Ingredients:

- 1 cup frozen pineapple chunks

- 1 teaspoon grated ginger

- Juice of 1 lime

- 1/2 cup unsweetened coconut milk

- 1/2 cup water

Instructions:

Add all ingredients to a blender and blend until smooth.

<u>**5. Pineapple Kale Smoothie:**</u>

This smoothie is high in antioxidants, which aid in the battle against cancer cells, and it is also low in calories, making it ideal for weight reduction.

Ingredients:

- 2 cups chopped kale leaves

- 1 cup frozen pineapple chunks

- 1/2 cup unsweetened almond milk

- 1/2 cup water

Instructions:

Add all ingredients to a blender and blend until smooth.

6. Peach Mango Smoothie:

Mangoes are high in vitamin C and antioxidants, which may help prevent cancer, whereas peaches are high in a range of vitamins and minerals that are beneficial to overall health.

Ingredients:

- 1 cup frozen mango chunks

- 1 medium peach, peeled and chopped

- Juice of 1/2 lime

- 1/2 cup unsweetened coconut milk

Instructions:

Add all ingredients to a blender and blend until smooth.

<u>**7. Papaya Carrot Smoothie:**</u>

Papaya includes enzymes that are supposed to suppress cancer cell development, but carrots are high in beta-carotene, which is turned into vitamin A in the body and is also thought to combat cancer.

Ingredients:

- 1 cup frozen papaya chunks

- 1 medium carrot, peeled and chopped

- 1/2 cup unsweetened coconut milk

- 1/2 cup water

Instructions:

Add all ingredients to a blender and blend until smooth.

8. Chocolate Berry Smoothie:

Dark chocolate includes antioxidants that have been found to lessen the incidence of some forms of cancer, whilst berries are high in vitamins and antioxidants that aid in cancer prevention.

Ingredients:

- 1 cup frozen mixed berries

- 1 tablespoon raw cacao powder

- 1/2 banana

- 1/2 cup unsweetened almond milk

Instructions:

Add all ingredients to a blender and blend until smooth.

9. Cherry Tomato Basil Smoothie:

Cherry tomatoes contain lycopene, a potent antioxidant linked to a decreased risk of cancer, and basil is a plant thought to have anti-cancer qualities.

Ingredients:

- 1 cup cherry tomatoes

- 1/4 cup fresh basil leaves

- 1/4 cup chopped red onion

- 1/2 cup unsweetened almond milk

- 1/2 cup water

Instructions:

Add all ingredients to a blender and blend until smooth.

10. Kiwi Pear Smoothie:

Both kiwi and pear are high in vitamins and antioxidants, which aid in cancer prevention and overall wellness.

Ingredients:

- 2 medium kiwis, peeled and chopped

- 1 medium pear, peeled and chopped

- Juice of 1/2 lemon

- 1/2 cup unsweetened almond milk

Instructions:

Add all ingredients to a blender and blend until smooth.

Before making any dietary changes, especially if you have a significant medical condition like cancer, you should check with your healthcare practitioner or a trained dietitian. The smoothie recipes in this extra chapter are meant to supplement, not replace, your entire cancer management approach.

Cancer is a complicated disease, and each case is different. What works for one individual might not work for the next. These recipes are intended to provide food and support, but they should not be used as a stand-alone treatment. It is essential to incorporate them into a well-balanced diet as well as a thorough healthcare routine customized to your unique requirements.

Some substances may also interfere with drugs or treatment methods. Your healthcare professional can advise you on whether these recipes are appropriate for your specific situation.

Incorporating Healthy Habits for Managing Fatty Liver Disease

Fatty liver disease is a significant health problem that, if not treated properly, can lead to difficulties. It is caused by an accumulation of fat in the liver and can be caused by a number of reasons such as obesity, high blood sugar levels, and excessive alcohol intake. There are, fortunately, things you can do to control your fatty liver disease and enhance your liver health.

Incorporating healthy behaviors into your everyday routine is one of the most crucial tasks.

Healthy Habit #1

Exercise Regularly

Exercise is a great strategy to enhance your liver health and lower your chance of getting fatty liver disease. Regular physical exercise helps to minimize liver inflammation, which can assist in avoiding injury and facilitate recovery.

Exercise also improves insulin sensitivity, which lowers the chance of developing non-alcoholic fatty liver disease.

Aim for at least 150 minutes of moderate aerobic activity each week to reap the maximum benefits from exercise. Physical activities such as brisk walking, swimming, and cycling are recommended. If you're beginning from scratch, start softly and gradually raise the intensity.

Healthy Habit #2

Mind Your Stress Levels

Excessive stress may also play a role in liver inflammation. When you are stressed, your body releases hormones that might induce liver inflammation and contribute to the advancement of fatty liver disease. You may alleviate stress by incorporating activities such as meditation, yoga, and deep breathing into your everyday routine. These hobbies can help you relax and lower your stress levels. Additionally, engaging in enjoyable activities can assist to relieve stress and produce a sense of calm. This might involve activities such as reading, drawing, or listening to music.

Healthy Habit #3

Maintain a Healthy Diet

Diet is critical in the management of fatty liver disease and liver health. A nutritious diet can help decrease inflammation and improve liver function. When it comes to fatty liver disease management, it is critical to minimize the consumption of items that might cause inflammation, such as fatty meats, processed meals, and sweets.

Instead, eat a diet strong in nutritious grains, fruits, vegetables, and lean protein. Grilled chicken with quinoa and roasted veggies is an example of a nutritious dinner.

Healthy Habit #4

Stay Hydrated

Water is essential for liver health because it keeps the liver functioning correctly. Furthermore, staying hydrated will help you maintain your energy levels and avoid weariness, which can be a side effect of fatty liver disease. Aim for at least eight to ten glasses of water every day. Reduce your intake of sugary beverages, such as energy drinks and soda, as they can lead to liver inflammation.

Healthy Habit #5

Get Enough Sleep

Sleep is essential for general health and well-being, and it is also critical for liver health. Getting adequate sleep might assist to minimize liver inflammation and facilitate recovery. Inadequate sleep, on the other hand, can aggravate fatty liver disease by contributing to inflammation.

Aim for 7-9 hours of peaceful sleep each night to ensure you're receiving plenty.

You may make crucial efforts to control fatty liver disease and enhance liver health by implementing these healthy practices into your daily routine. Start small, since little changes can lead to major gains in your general health and well-being over time. Remember, the goal is to remain persistent and to include these good behaviors in your daily routine.

Frequently Asked Questions

It is natural for someone suffering from fatty liver disease to have questions about their condition and the role that juicing can play in improving their liver health. Here are some of the most frequently asked questions, along with accurate and informative answers.

Section 1: Common Concerns about Juicing and Fatty Liver Disease

1. Is it safe for me to juice if I have fatty liver disease?

Yes! In fact, juicing is a great way to get more fruits and vegetables into your diet, which can help reduce inflammation and promote liver function. Just make sure to eat low-sugar, high-nutrient fruits and vegetables like kale, spinach, beets, and berries.

2. Will juicing assist me in losing weight and improving my fatty liver disease?

Yes, it is possible! Juicing can be a quick and easy way to consume more fruits and vegetables while reducing your consumption of processed foods and sugary beverages. This can aid in weight loss, which can lead to an improvement in fatty liver disease.

3. Should I avoid drinking fruit juice if I have fatty liver disease?

No, not always. While it is important to limit your consumption of sugary beverages, you can still include fruit juices in your diet as long as they are made from whole fruits and do not contain added sugars. Just make sure to choose low-sugar, high-nutrient fruits like berries, citrus fruits, and apples.

Section 2: Addressing Misconceptions and Myths

1. Is moderate alcohol consumption beneficial to my liver?

No, any amount of alcohol can be harmful to your liver, especially if you have fatty liver disease. Alcohol is processed by your liver, which can cause inflammation and cell damage, leading to fatty liver disease and other complications.

2. Is a low-carbohydrate diet the best way to manage fatty liver disease?

No, not always. While a low-carb diet may be beneficial for some people, it is critical to focus on a well-balanced diet rich in fruits and vegetables, lean protein, and whole grains. These foods are beneficial to liver health because they help to reduce inflammation and promote healing.

3. Can juicing alone cure my fatty liver disease?

While juicing can help with fatty liver disease management, it is not a cure. Fatty liver disease is best managed with a mix of lifestyle modifications, such as exercise and a balanced diet, and medical therapy when needed.

Finally, as long as you focus on nutrient-dense fruits and vegetables and avoid additional sweets, juicing can be a safe and effective strategy to control fatty liver disease. Remember that the best method to manage fatty liver disease is a mix of lifestyle modifications and medical therapy, so talk to your doctor about your symptoms and the best course of action for you.

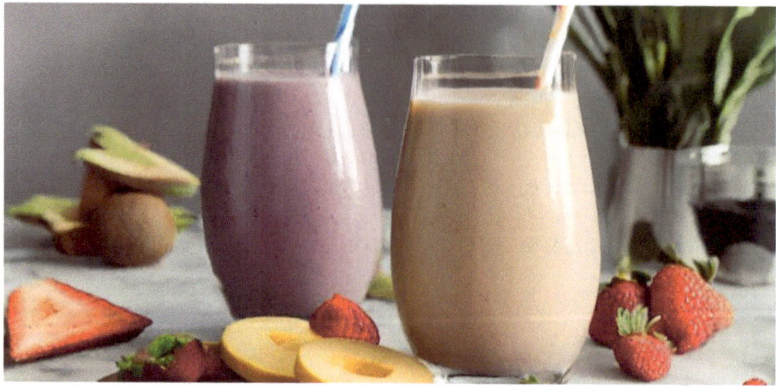

Conclusion: Juicing for Fatty Liver – A Path towards Health

Thank you for making it to the end of this book, which is a significant first step in treating your fatty liver condition. In this book, we've looked at how juicing may help improve liver health and reduce inflammation, as well as the most nutritious fruits and vegetables to juice for this reason.

But, more importantly, I hope this book has given you a sense of optimism and empowerment. Fatty liver disease can be a frightening and daunting diagnosis, but by changing your food and lifestyle, you are actively trying to restore your body and improve your long-term health.

Juicing into your daily routine provides your body with a concentrated dosage of vitamins, minerals, and antioxidants that can help decrease inflammation and support liver function. However, juicing is not a cure-all, and it's important to remember that the most effective method to manage fatty liver disease is through a mix of lifestyle modifications and medical therapy as prescribed by your healthcare professional.

Finally, I'd want to thank you for taking the time to read this book and for taking charge of your own health. Keep in mind that you are not alone on this trip, and that there are tools and assistance available to you as you proceed. If you found this book useful, I recommend that you look at my other works on fatty liver disease and related issues.

Remember that you are capable of making great changes in your life, and that investing in your health and well-being is worthwhile. You may find your own unique road to health and recovery with the correct tools and a commitment to study and grow.

Thank you for purchasing and reading this book. I sincerely hope that you have found the solution to your problem in the pages of this book. If you have enjoyed reading this book, please leave a kind review so others can find the book and also get the help they need.

Also below, are a books you will enjoy reading.

- **The Plant-Based Fatty Liver Diet Cookbook** - 100+ Recipes to Help You Lose Weight, Improve Your Liver Health, and Feel Your Best *Bonus – 12 Exciting Plant Based Dessert Recipes to Satisfy Your Sweet tooth Cravings!*

- **"The Quick and Easy Ketogenic Diet for Women Over 60"** - The Ultimate Solution to Achieving a Healthy and Vibrant Lifestyle with Quick, Convenient Great-Tasting, Low-carb Keto Recipes *Bonus - 7-Day Green Smoothie Meal Plan for Active Women Above 60 worth $6.69*

- **A Fatty Liver Diet Breakfast Cookbook:** Explore 20 Delicious Quick and Easy Recipes to Regain Energy, Detox, Loose Weight, and Revitalize Your Liver

- **Heart-healthy cooking with DASH** - 215 Delicious Recipes For Managing High Blood Pressure Naturally *Bonus – 20 Heart-Healthy Smoothie Recipes*

All titles are available on Amazon.